C*The* aregiver's
TAO TE CHING

T0126152

The Caregiver's
TAO TE CHING

COMPASSIONATE CARING FOR
YOUR LOVED ONES AND YOURSELF

William and Nancy Martin

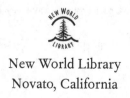

New World Library
Novato, California

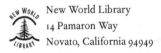 New World Library
14 Pamaron Way
Novato, California 94949

The material in this book is intended for education. It is not meant to take the place
of diagnosis and treatment by a qualified medical practitioner or therapist. No expressed or implied guarantee as to the effects of the use of the recommendations
can be given nor liability taken.

Text design by Tona Pearce Myers

Sumi-e brush illustrations by ~freak76 at http://freak76.deviantart.com/art/
Sumi-e-brushes-49605766

Library of Congress Cataloging-in-Publication Data
Martin, William, date.
 The caregiver's Tao te ching : compassionate caring for your loved ones and yourself / William and Nancy Martin.
    p.   cm.
 ISBN 978-1-57731-888-0 (pbk. : alk. paper)
 1. Care of the sick—Religious aspects—Taoism—Meditations. I. Martin, Nancy,
date. II. Title.
BL1942.8.M37 2011
299.5'14432—dc22   2010041981

First printing, January 2011
ISBN 978-1-57731-888-0
Printed in Canada on 100% postconsumer-waste recycled paper

New World Library is a proud member of the Green Press Initiative.

10 9 8 7 6 5 4 3 2

To Betty Ann Elliott, who let us share her life and death and who demonstrated the Tao of grace and courage

[CONTENTS]

[ACKNOWLEDGMENTS]

WE ARE DEEPLY GRATEFUL for all the people who touch our lives in extraordinary ways.

We are grateful for Barbara Moulton, our agent, who first suggested this book. She has been our guide and friend and has responded to our hopes and fears with patience and wisdom.

We are grateful for Jason Gardner, our editor, and Mimi Kusch, our copy editor, who worked with us to clearly communicate the power of the caregiving experience.

We are grateful for the community of wonderful people who practice Zen with us at the Still Point. They have shown us the true nature of compassionate awareness.

We are grateful for each other. Our life together has been a gift of priceless value.

ACKNOWLEDGMENTS

[INTRODUCTION]

Our Journey

We began this book to express our gratitude for the wisdom and encouragement that the classic Chinese text the *Tao Te Ching* has brought to us over the past twenty years. Its author, Lao Tzu, though a legendary figure from 2,600 years ago, feels like a trusted elder uncle, watching us with compassion and acceptance as we have walked, skipped, and stumbled along the paths of our lives. His understanding of how the Tao expresses itself in every atom of the cosmos has helped us maintain our balance through all the seasons of our life together: our love for each other, our relationship with our children, and our acceptance of our own aging. In *The Caregiver's Tao Te Ching*, we hope to craft some of Lao Tzu's wisdom, especially for those who find themselves, willingly or not, in the role of caregiver.

Life does not unfold according to our wishes. It is not predictable. It does not follow a smooth and comfortable path. It offers beauty and love mixed with transience and loss, creating a marvelous melancholy — a blend of pleasure and pain that brings intensity and mystery to existence. In the midst of such complexity, the ability to give care to one another is an essential part of a meaningful and compassionate life.

We started this book almost two years ago because we felt that our combined experience would allow us to offer support to those in professional or personal caregiving situations. Nancy had spent eleven years as a minister specializing in life transitions. She also had spent five years working for Enloe Hospice in Chico, California, training and supporting volunteers who gave practical, emotional, and spiritual support to hundreds of dying people and their families. She then started her own independent intensive training program, Zen Compassionate Care, which used a foundation of Zen awareness practice to develop caregiving skills. Bill brought thirty years of experience as a counselor, teacher, and Taoist scholar/author. We felt professionally competent and ready to write the book. Now, as we finish the book two years later, we have a new and far more personal perspective.

About a year ago we moved into an apartment near Nancy's ninety-year-old mother, Betty Ann. Betty Ann was slowing down but cherished her independent life in her sunny second-floor apartment and wanted to remain there. We moved into the same complex so that we could check in on her as part of our daily rhythm.

In late summer 2009, Betty Ann's congestive heart failure began to usher her from one stage of letting go to the next, and Nancy's caregiving moved from the professional and theoretical to the personal and intense. In September Betty Ann could no longer safely live alone, so Nancy began sleeping in a twin bed beside her, helping her remain oriented during wakeful periods at night.

Betty Ann continued to let go — of walking on her own, of sitting up, finally of eating. With the support of a wonderful hospice team, Nancy maintained her position as director of the Still Point Zen Center yet spent most of her time at her mother's side, watching and helping as she could. On December 11, after a wakeful night trying to help Betty Ann find a comfortable position for breathing, Nancy sat by her bed for her morning meditation. Nancy could see a large, bare tree just outside the window. As she began to meditate, a hawk came to rest on a limb of the tree, looking in the window. As Nancy let her breath settle and become slow and regular she noticed that Betty Ann's breath had settled into the same rhythm. Throughout the thirty-minute meditation they breathed at the same gentle pace, and the hawk remained motionless in the tree. At the close of meditation, Nancy stood, bowed to her mother, and turned and bowed to the hawk. The hawk flew away, and Betty Ann let go of her last breath. It felt like she had joined him in flight

It would have been easier to write this book from a detached position, giving advice from safe ground. But the ever-changing energy of the Tao took a different expression. The final touches of the book have had to emerge as Nancy grieved her mother's death and settled her affairs. The emotions are still tender. The fatigue is still heavy.

It is our deepest hope that the ancient wisdom of Lao Tzu, which pours through the Tao, will join with our present-day direct experience of tenderness and loss to express the true nature of giving and receiving care. At the core of our being lies an ancient, innate wisdom. This is the source and power of compassionate care. It allows each of us to live out this task in our own unique way.

Your caregiving journey may be similar to ours, or it may be quite different. You may be helping a loved one through recovery from an illness or surgery. You may be caring for someone with a long-term disability. You may be called to give care in one or more of hundreds of different ways. Whatever your situation, you will benefit from the support of Lao Tzu's wisdom and from an awareness of your own deep connection with the essence of life that he called the Tao.

The Chinese character for *Tao* has many possible translations. It can simply mean "path," as in a path to your front door, or it can refer to many different types of ways and paths. Lao Tzu used the character in its most expansive sense — the mysterious Way in which the cosmos unfolds itself. He uses the character *Te* to refer to the energy and power with which this Tao operates. So his book the *Tao Te Ching* literally means "The Book of the Way and Its Power."

The *Tao Te Ching* is not a linear book. It does not present a tightly organized scheme of premises and conclusions. Instead, it is a collection of poems, each touching on one of the characteristics of the Tao that can be observed as it manifests itself. It often repeats themes, visiting them from different angles. It can be inspiring, confusing, and frustrating for those of us with the Western habit of wanting answers spelled out clearly.

Caregiving is much the same. It does not unfold in an orderly fashion. It evades easy answers. We would like to wrap it up in neat bundles of conclusions we can rely on, but it refuses to remain tidy and orderly. It is sometimes gratifying, often frustrating, always a mystery.

Caregiving and the Tao have other characteristics in common. Each asks that we show up and have a direct experience of life as it is unfolding in this moment. Each seems unpredictable to our conditioned mind yet follows its own course and asks us to follow along. Each contains paradoxes that our desires and opinions cannot resolve and therefore asks for our acceptance. Each asks not for a grand plan but for a willingness to take the next simple step.

Two Minds

We use the terms *conditioned mind* and *Tao mind* to describe the two basic perspectives from which we human beings can experience life. Our conditioned mind is the conscious sense of identity we have learned through a lifetime of input from our parents, friends, culture, and events. This identity is a natural function of the brain and allows us to make reasonable decisions about what actions to take in any given circumstance.

But conditioned mind is too narrow and limited to serve as the only locus of self-identity. We believe that there is a deeper, broader, unconditioned sense of identity and perspective, which we call Tao mind. From this perspective we do not see ourselves as separate from all that is happening. Here our intuition and natural wisdom are available, unrestricted by the learned beliefs, opinions, and fears that dominate so much of our lives and so easily contaminate our caregiving.

Your own experience of caregiving can be a unique opportunity to live from the perspective of the Tao, from your own Tao mind. This will be quite a different way of seeing life and may seem frightening and strange at times. Be assured that you are completely capable of this experience and that it will, in fact, begin to usher you into an awareness and freedom that will transform your life.

In a sense, there is only one message of Lao Tzu's book and therefore of ours: "You are, by nature, an expression of the Tao, and its wisdom and power are part of your true nature. Let go of the stories to the contrary and live in wonder and appreciation." Lao Tzu called attention to this message from many different angles, but it remained the core of his teaching. Each caregiving situation is unique in many ways, but the essence of effective and compassionate response remains the same. Lao Tzu used only five thousand words to express this. We have used almost four times that many, but we have tried to keep to the same essential theme. Lao Tzu repeated his basic themes often, offering a slightly different vantage point each time. We have tried to do the same. Each element of the book is an invitation to look once again, gently, compassionately, and with deep acceptance at what is arising in you. No matter how complex the details of your situation, what you truly desire and need is that basic trust in life, in the Tao, and in yourself. This is the message of every chapter. Let it sink deep into your awareness.

We offer you all our tender wishes. You can contact us through our website, www.thestillpoint.com. Don't hesitate to write and share your journey with us. We know the hopes and fears you face, and we deeply care.

[I]
Let Go

Caring for loved ones with your ideas
and caring for them with your actions
are two different processes.
The first arises within your mind
and often brings confusion.
The second is a direct experience,
free of mental voices,
and leads to clarity.

The mind that wants to help
does not know how.
The mind that lets go of wanting
knows exactly what to do.
Both minds reside within us.
Learning to live with both
unlocks the secret of caregiving.

Be quietly present with yourself
in the presence of another human being.
If you can do this you will know
the next simple thing to do.
This is all that is ever necessary.

THE FIRST STEP IN CAREGIVING is to let go of our ideas about
what it means to be a helpful, compassionate caregiver. These
mental images set standards that easily lead to disappoint-
ment, frustration, and self-doubt. The direct experience of
giving care is new every moment and leads us in unfamiliar

directions. We gather experience along the way, but with each encounter we must show up, stay present to what is actually happening, and see what occurs. When we do this, a space opens in which compassion for everyone involved, including ourselves, can naturally arise.

Caring for another person is not about orchestrating the tasks of the day so that we can do it "right." It is about letting go of our ideas and making room for the two people who are here in this place, in this moment. It is the freedom to be who we are and to open our hearts to ourselves and to those in our care.

Come and Go

You cannot give another person
happiness without sadness,
comfort without pain,
gain without loss,
or life without death.
Do not try.

Let your helping be without agenda.
Let the natural course of things unfold.
Do what you do,
and think no more about it.
This will bring freedom
to giver and receiver alike.

LIFE IS A RICH MIXTURE OF SENSATIONS, emotions, ideas, and experiences. They arise, build, and then ebb at their own pace. As much as we long to cling to the positive experiences and avoid the painful, all experiences come and go as part of life.

When we resist the sensations or emotions of the moment we create suffering. Now we face not just physical discomfort but also the internal judgment that our feelings are wrong, unfair, and unendurable.

We care for our loved ones with the intention of adding to their comfort and lessening their pain. Yet there are days when neither can be accomplished. The experience of the day is not what we wanted for ourselves or for the one in our care. Freedom comes as we do what seems best in the moment and simply let the outcome be what it is. Without review or evaluation we can simply let life reveal the next natural step.

[3]

Acceptance Brings Change

Clinging to how we think things should be
brings confusion and despair.
Seeing things be as they are
brings clarity.
Clarity leads to effective action.

Trying to change others
leads to resistance and frustration.
Seeing others as they are
leads to acceptance.
Acceptance leads to change.

TO ACCEPT WHAT IS HAPPENING in this moment, this situation, this season of life, does not require us to like it. Acceptance is the simple act of acknowledging what is true — this sensation, this fear, this frustration, or this dread that we are experiencing right now. Avoiding it only adds sorrow and suffering to what is already painful.

It takes courage to step forward into the reality of the moment. This person who is dear to our heart is weak, ill, injured, recovering slowly, or dying. She will experience a whole range of responses as symptoms change and she moves from hope to despair, from resignation to peace.

We are here to share this life as it is, one moment at a time. Acceptance is the first step in becoming a true companion in this journey. It will bring the clarity and openness that will reveal what is possible now.

[4]

Inexhaustible Source

Striving, we become exhausted.
Ceasing to strive, we find astonishing energy.
Tranquility rests within us,
softening our edges
and bringing us peace.

Where does it come from?
Someplace we can't name.
What is its source?
Something inexhaustible.
What does it do?
Everything that needs to be done.

WE HAVE BEEN TAUGHT not to trust our true nature and to look outside ourselves for peace, tranquility, and wisdom. Yet at the core of who we are lies an ancient, innate wisdom. This is our natural connection with the Tao.

This connection is called by many names. We talk of returning to our "own hearts" or coming back to "center." We speak of our "true nature," which is compassion. In all these ways we point to something that cannot be named. It can only be rediscovered through direct experience.

We recognize it when we are doing well in the midst of the challenges of caregiving. We see it when we know deep within that all truly is well, even in the middle of the most distressing day. We sense it when we find tenderness welling up to soothe our frustration and despair when we feel we are failing at our task.

Watch for these experiences. They are available to all of us, to remind us of the trustworthiness of our own hearts.

[5]
Sitting Quietly

Expecting life to bring us what we want
and to deliver us from what we do not want
is to suffer needlessly.
Finding that we are adequate
for everything that happens
is to be at peace.

Preferring some things
and avoiding others,
we struggle through life.
Sitting quietly and breathing deeply,
we find renewal within ourselves.
Sitting quietly with another person,
we watch him find renewal
within himself.

SITTING QUIETLY IN MEDITATION we practice opening our
hearts to whatever arises within. We do not abandon ourselves, no matter what sensations, thoughts, or moods arise.
No longer believing that we must escape the intensity of our
inner experience, we stay right with the sensations as they
arise, peak, and then ebb. We rest in the breath, feeling it as it
moves into and out of the body. Its rhythm reminds us to take
in this vivid moment of life and then let it go.

As we become more at ease with all the intensity that
flows through our beings, we find that we can remain present
with what is happening. In this way we build proof that we
can endure and even welcome all that life presents, one moment at a time.

[6]

Hidden, but Never Absent

You cannot give another person joy,
for joy has never left her.
It is what is always there
beneath the struggles and the pain,
hidden,
but never absent.

You cannot make another person see it.
You can only see it for yourself.
The more you see it in all things,
the more she sees it in herself.

THE TASKS OF CAREGIVING can distract us from the joy that
endures even in the most difficult situations. We become lost
in responding to symptoms, complaints, and needs. We forget
that this person is not a problem to be solved but someone we
deeply care for.

When we sink below the surface demands, the joy of
being part of one another's life remains. A gruff father soft-
ens and at moments takes on a childlike glow. A child who has
been struggling with pain finds a moment of delight as something makes her laugh. A frail mother gets the giggles as she
tries to find her elusive balance halfway between sitting and
standing. This joy finds ways to bubble up to the surface at
unexpected moments. We do not need to create it or make it
appear. It will emerge on its own. We just notice and savor it.

[7]
Room to Work

How can we reveal to another person
the mysterious comfort of the eternal Tao?

By seeing without judgment
and listening without interpreting.
By waiting without purpose
and sharing without agenda.

In this way we become an empty space,
not cluttered with our own perceptions.
In this space the Tao has room to work.

THE PERSON WE ARE CARING FOR is in the midst of a complex process. So are we. Part of what we can offer is the compassionate space needed to contain all that is happening. A helpful image is of a large, shallow, empty bowl that occupies the space between us and the one in our care. Into this bowl the care receiver can pour out anything and everything.

We listen without comments or advice. We take nothing personally as he shares, so there is no limit to what he can pour out in our presence. We reflect back a few of his own words to help him continue untangling the jumble of thoughts and emotions that come as his body no longer behaves as it once did.

It is not up to us to find or give answers. In this safe place, the one in our care will find those answers emerging in his own words.

[8]
Clarity

The Tao flows like water
into all the nooks and crannies of life,
nurturing everything without distinction.
As water lets the nature of the terrain
determine its course,
so the Tao lets circumstances
determine its actions.

This is how we do our work:
not assuming what is needed
but letting the moment determine our actions;
not withholding our intrinsic goodness
but giving nurture wherever it is needed;
not pushing forcefully ahead
but waiting patiently for clarity to emerge.

A RIVER YIELDS TO THE CHANGING FEATURES in the riverbed that holds it. Nothing is truly an obstacle as the water continues its inevitable movement, finding the course that the Tao provides. In our caregiving we do not know what will happen from one day to the next or even over the next few hours. If we cling to assumptions and plans we can feel thrown off balance by the unexpected. We end up bracing ourselves and feel separate from the flow of the Tao.

Yet we are never separate from life's unfolding. When we trust this deep reality, we find ourselves once again in harmony with the Tao. Our intrinsic goodness guides us to the next simple thing to do. What is truly nurturing in this moment will make itself clear.

[9]

Because We Want To

Wanting gratitude for our actions,
we are never satisfied.
Trying to control the situation,
we are never secure.
Looking for approval,
we are never happy.

If we do what we do
just because we want to,
the doing itself is all we will ever need.

OUR CHILDHOOD EXPERIENCES naturally condition us to look for approval and to feel safe when we receive it. The smiles and frowns of parents and teachers train us to look to others to see if we are doing things well and if we are loved and accepted. This desire for approval is naturally present in our caregiving experience as well.

Trusting the Tao in our caregiving, we find that our fulfillment is not dependent on someone else's response. When we become aware of searching for external signs of approval or disapproval, we can gently lay it aside. The satisfaction we truly desire comes from recognizing our willingness to care for another person, regardless of his or her response. We are doing this because we want to.

[10]
Soft and Tender

Can you take caring action
yet remain centered in your body
and never lose your soul?
Can you remain soft and tender
without trying to control?
Can you wait patiently
without feeling helpless?
Can you love
and not possess?
This is the way of the Tao.

This ability is naturally ours.
Caring and tenderness arise
from who we truly are.
Patience and love
are waiting in our hearts.
We are the way of the Tao as well.

PROVIDING CARE PUSHES US INTO SITUATIONS we would usually avoid. The intensity of the emotions it stirs can make us want to flee. While at any other time we would withdraw to escape this discomfort, now we choose to remain.

It is a perfect time to discover our own depth. We are pushed to let go of our efforts to control life and to protect our self-image of being calm and collected. Instead we must sink into our own hearts to find the tenderness, softness, and vulnerability that will sustain us.

When we become tender, we find room to breathe and acceptance of who we are. Our muscles can relax, and our soul can find rest. It is this soft and loving way that will see us through all that caregiving brings.

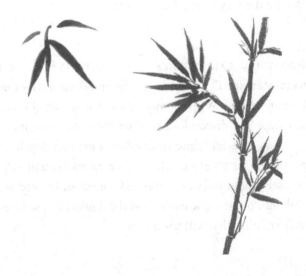

[11]

Spaciousness

How do we stay balanced
on the ever-turning wheel of change?
By moving to the center
and letting the wheel spin as it will.
By remaining empty,
making room for all the feelings that arise
in ourselves and others.

The myriad events of whirling life
are the materials of our work.
The spaciousness within
is where the work is done.

WE ARE TAUGHT TO BE CREATURES OF HABIT. We develop routines and schedules to move through the day without noticing what we are doing. We prefer patterns in providing care that allow us to feel confident and at ease. Our conditioned mind prefers to be on automatic pilot, unruffled by the specifics of life.

The ever-changing nature of life invites us to pay attention. Yesterday our hand on her back as she rose from her chair was just a symbol of support. Today we both feel the difference. Her arms shake with the effort, and she needs a boost to get to her feet. Tomorrow her legs may be stronger after a good night's rest, but they may not be. Either way, the changes will continue to come.

Compassionate awareness creates room for all the hopes, fears, sorrows, and uncertainties to well up and then subside.

Supported from within, we do not need to make life stop spinning around us. The Tao provides refuge in the midst of it all, where both of us are safe just as we are.

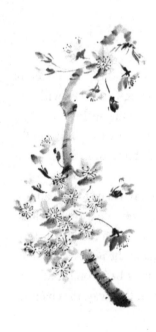

[12]

The Tao Is Silent

Our conditioned mind tells itself scary stories
to keep itself stirred up.
It looks for amusements
to keep itself distracted.
It creates problems
to keep itself busy.
Given its way
it would never let us rest.
It is the source of every fear.

Our Tao mind is silent.
Thus it is the source
of every loving action.

CONDITIONED MIND IS THE LIFELONG ACCUMULATION of mental habits that we develop to protect ourselves from pain, uncertainty, and danger. Its task is to keep us living within the safe confines of the familiar and comfortable.

Whenever we step outside this narrow box, our conditioned mind roars up with all the reasons why we must escape these unwanted feelings and experiences. This reel of commentary in our minds offers us every option except that of being fully present.

Tao mind knows that we are never separate from life and that we do not need to be. It points to the direct experience of each moment. It sees circumstances as they are. It does not add fearful commentary that clouds our vision. From the clear, compassionate perspective of Tao mind, loving action naturally emerges.

Neither Praise nor Blame

Be wary of both praise and blame.
Our conditioned mind will use them
to keep us fearful
and unable to see clearly what to do.
It will praise us for taking care of a person in need,
then blame us for not doing it well enough.
It will keep us constantly off balance,
always concerned with "how we're doing."

Praise feels good for a moment,
so we tend to seek it.
Blame feels uncomfortable,
so we try to avoid it.
Our Tao mind will ignore the commentaries
and do whatever comes its way to do
with full attention and freedom.

PRAISE AND BLAME are not part of the natural flow of life. They are arbitrary standards imposed after the fact for reviewing and evaluating what has already happened. Whether the source of praise and blame is another person or our inner critic, we end up measuring our thoughts and actions against vague and shifting standards of "how we ought to be." When we believe that they can guide our life, we abandon trust in our innate wisdom and look for outside clues to see if we are measuring up.

When we return to our Tao mind, no commentary is needed. Our words and actions emerge naturally as we move through the day. When what we try does not work out the way we had hoped, we seek the next possibility. When things flow smoothly, we enjoy the feeling of living in harmony with the Tao. There is no praise or blame. There is only the unconditional freedom to let one experience inform the next.

The Source of All Caring

What motivates a caregiver's actions?
Why are we willing to be with another's pain?
Who can say?
We want to help,
but that's not the whole story.
We feel obliged,
but that's not it either.
Beneath the many motives of the conditioned mind
rests the mysterious Tao,
which is the true source of all caring.
We can't see it or understand it.
We can only trust that it
is the origin of what we do
and the power that helps us see it through.

WHEN WE ENTER A CAREGIVING RELATIONSHIP, we may think we are doing so for all the usual reasons. We are the nearest family member or the one who has always gotten along best with our aging parent. Caregiving is our dearest passion, or it is the career we have chosen. These reasons are enough to bring us to this task, but they are not strong enough to carry us through it.

A much deeper life current has brought us to caregiving — the courage, compassion, and wisdom of our heart that have always longed for expression. We are here to discover the deep heroic service we are capable of giving. We are here to uncover the quiet patience of our soul that has always longed to celebrate the fullness of another person's life.

At the heart of our caring is the willingness to be more vulnerable and therefore more fully alive than ever before. This is the power that keeps us returning day by day to the ever-changing journey of caregiving.

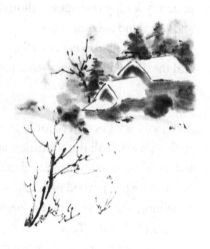

As a Guest

What would it be like to give care
while centered in the Tao?

We would pay attention to everything
but get caught up in nothing.
We would be alert
but never tense.
We would be like a guest in another's life
and remain in the background.
We would not manipulate our host
but remain patient,
waiting until "what to do" does itself.
We would be like a valley that welcomes the river
and whatever else comes.

To do this we must sit and wait,
patiently letting our muddy thoughts settle
and our mind become clear.
Awareness will become our ally,
and the Tao will be our companion.

AT TIMES WE SINK INTO OUR CONNECTION with the Tao in such a way that all the confusion and tension fade away. The voices of our conditioned mind take on a tissue-paper quality, because we live beyond their reach. The question of being able or willing to provide care no longer holds any meaning. We are centered in the Tao.

From our own center come a calm watching and listening.

None of this is about us. It is entirely the experience of those in our care. We are here to provide quiet companionship through territory that only they can see.

Our attention now rests on noticing the clues they give about what they need. There is no need to figure things out. We are a guest in their life. They will show us what is next.

Return to the Source

One change gets piled on top of another,
and we lose our balance.
One thought leads to another,
and we forget our Source.
This Source is at the center
of this spinning wheel of life.
It is the womb from which we came,
the home in which we live,
and the haven to which we journey.

As we return to this Source
our obsessive thoughts fade to silence
and our fear gives way to trust.

IN PROVIDING CARE we often experience a tumbling sensation as we respond to rapid changes. By the time we find a good solution, the situation has changed again. We are left scrambling, trying to keep up. We feel separate from life and helpless to regain the control and certainty we desperately desire.

This is a familiar cycle of suffering. Part of us really believes that we should know how to gracefully handle situations we have never encountered before. We lose sleep believing that we can anticipate the needs that will emerge tomorrow.

When we let go of this conditioned pattern, we can return to our Source — our own heart. Caregiving is not about solving every problem or knowing every answer. It is about trusting our innate wisdom and compassion, which remain steadfast through all the changes.

Hardly Even Noticed

Some caregivers are resented
because of their need to control.
Others are appreciated for all they do.
Others are loved.
But the Tao is hardly even noticed.

When we are free from our need to control,
from our need to be appreciated or loved,
those who receive our care
retain their own power
and remain the host of their own lives.

OUR CARE RECEIVER SHOULD NOT BEAR THE BURDEN of our good intentions. She should not use her energy defending herself against our good ideas and helpful advice. If she does, we have failed in the true task of supporting her journey.

Guided by the Tao, we enter gently into the flow of another person's experience. There is no hurry and no agenda to fulfill. We are here to offer a professional skill, a technique to simplify life, or gentle companionship.

Our first step is to see what new options she has discovered on her own. Has she already found an easier way to get out of bed or developed a plan to reduce the number of trips she makes across the room? Can we offer our energy in support of these new ways to do daily tasks rather than imposing our own ideas?

When we can, we are serving her innate wisdom and nurturing her independence. As she directs our actions, she may hardly notice that we are helping at all.

Depth, Not Duty

Caregiving must arise
from the depths of the heart.
If these depths are not tapped,
ideas such as "duty" and "loyalty"
take their place.

When duty and loyalty are exalted,
true caregiving disappears.
These things are an empty shell
and not adequate for meeting the challenge
of life's unwelcome changes.

THE WORDS *duty* and *loyalty* are fraught with conditioned meanings. The connotations are of remaining as aloof and untouched as possible while bravely doing what is expected. Suddenly obeying or disobeying, resisting or complying, becomes part of the process. All the assumptions and projections only add suffering to the situation.

Living by the wisdom of our heart, we have an entirely different experience. We are living out our basic compassion as we serve as another's companion. It is the nature of an open heart to be tender. In this gentle, accepting environment mutual trust can grow. We do not face the challenges of this time in isolation, holding to our designated tasks. We are in this together, growing in our compassionate caregiving relationship.

Compassionate Awareness

Trying to be kind, we end up interfering.
Trying to be helpful, we end up tinkering,
pushing, and generally being of no help at all.

True kindness appears when our true nature
touches the true nature of another person.
True helpfulness appears
when we are both simply together in the moment.
At this point we share the feeling
of compassionate awareness.

ON THE SURFACE we and the one in our care most likely have
very different perspectives on what it means to give and receive care. What we assume would be helpful feels threaten-
ing or disempowering to him. What he assumes we should
know without asking would never occur to us. If we remain
at this place, we bounce off of each other, and our frustration
grows. We are both trying hard but not accomplishing anything of value.

Sinking below the surface we find common ground. We
find that at heart we are the same. Both of us carry wisdom,
compassion, tenderness, and the desire to find a way through
the challenges.

Trusting this fundamental connection, we no longer look
at the situation or each other as things to be figured out. We
will grow in our understanding of each other as we share in
the mystery that is unfolding between us.

You Remain

Don't waste your time trying to understand
why things are as they are.
Don't believe all the stories you are told
about what's important
and not important.
Don't get stirred up by wanting this
and avoiding that.

You are a plain and simple being,
an expression of the Tao.
Even when everything you thought secure
is slipping out from under you,
you remain.

FOR MANY CAREGIVERS there comes a time of despair, a time
when we feel we have come to the end of our rope. The fatigue
and the endless need to adjust convince us that we just cannot
do it anymore. We feel that we have failed and that what we
thought was bedrock is crumbling beneath our feet.

In truth, we have not come to the end of our capacity for
life. When we finally give up and fall into this abyss, we find
that we fall into freedom.

It is not our basic nature that has crumbled, but the story
of who we have to be and how we have to act. When all that
falls away, we find the amazing wonder of who we have always
been. The letting go that we had been convinced would bring
ruin and shame instead brings freedom and deep gratitude for
the riches of our true nature.

True Nature

When you see everything changing
before your eyes,
have confidence in what you cannot see.
You cannot see the dance of energy
that forms the cosmos,
yet it fills all of space.
You cannot see the bonding forces
that knit your body into being,
yet you are here.
You cannot see your own true nature,
yet like the Tao it is ever present.
It is what is reading these words
at this moment,
here and now.
This is what you can trust.

WHAT CATCHES OUR ATTENTION so often dismays us. We see illness, infirmity, and injury, which seem to define our situation completely. We become wholly focused on the details of providing care and managing the symptoms of the body. It can become difficult to trust that anything exists beyond these realities.

Yet this body has been part of a dance since before the beginning of beginningless time. This dance is expressed in all the functions of organs and cells, emotions and thoughts that move through this being without any conscious effort from us.

Our trust lies not in being able to control the surface signs and symptoms. Beyond our sight, all things are still changing and evolving just as they always have. When we are still and listen to our heart, we know that we can trust this timeless, mysterious unfolding of living and dying. It is as amazing now as it was on the day we were born.

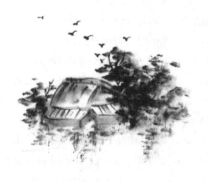

22

Refuge in What Is

Life feels crooked
when we want it straight,
and empty
when we want it full.
We sometimes get what we desire.
We sometimes lose
that which is most precious to us.
The future cannot be predicted,
and therefore it frightens us.

Taking refuge in what is,
we find relief from all our struggle.
No longer demanding something different,
we find a simple peace within.
Not trying to control events,
we preserve our energy.
We are no longer in opposition to life
so our strength is fully available
and our spirit is capable of all that is needed.

MANY OF US WERE RAISED TO BELIEVE that if we do everything right we can avoid pain, fear, and sorrow. We grow up believing that the unwanted experiences of life are beyond our strength to endure. We think that we must keep them at bay, or life will be too much for us.

The reality is that these challenges prove what has always been true: life *is* beyond our control. It does not yield to our preferences or shield us from our fears. The moment may come when the certainty of death and our helplessness to do anything about it will flood us with a mixture of terror and awe.

Faced with this inescapable truth, we find the courage to allow people to become precious to us. We can allow ourselves to sink into the vulnerability of our heart and to feel the sadness and grief, the sweetness and sorrow that naturally flow through these days.

Nestled in this deep, rich melancholy of life, we can remain fully available to the one in our care. Far from being beyond enduring, life finds room for everything in a heart opened wide.

Everything Has Its Time

The strongest winds wreak havoc
but die away with time.
The rain may last for weeks
but finally passes over.
Even the cosmos
will finally pass away.
Everything has its time.
Everything passes.

If we open ourselves to life
we become one with all we are
and with all we do.
Joy and sorrow become part
of just one wondrous whole.
Within this whole,
everything has its time.

BEING FULLY PRESENT as those in our care struggle with their feelings of helplessness, pain, sorrow, resentment, uncertainty, gratitude, and love will feel like watching a series of storms blowing through. The sensations that arise in our bodies as we watch and listen will reveal our own deepest beliefs, fears, joys, and assumptions about life.

As we become more confident that we are capable of everything we experience, we discover that those we care for are also capable of all this intensity. From our own experience we know that all feelings, moods, and thoughts are transient. They all appear, grow, manifest in their fullness, and ebb.

Whether it is anger, fear, sadness, frustration, wonder, or a wild mixture of them all, it will have its own life span and then slowly disappear.

Remembering this, we do not have to flee strong emotions or try to change the mood of our care receivers. We are not here to keep the storms away but to be a calm presence as the whirlwinds blow on through. When the storm has passed, we will both rest.

It Happened by Itself

All our striving seems to push away
the very peace we are seeking.
We grasp for hope,
and it eludes us.
We stretch for safety,
and it remains evasive.

When we cease striving
and stop grasping and stretching,
we find that we are carried by the Tao.
What we tried to accomplish by our efforts
we find has happened by itself.

WHEN WE REACT TO THE UNKNOWN with tension and urgency, we can find ourselves perched at the edge of the chair, leaning forward toward life. Caught up in this tight vigilance we anticipate potential needs and grasp at small signs of improvement. This physical and mental tension leaves us exhausted, frustrated, discouraged, and lost.

When we become aware of these feelings, we can choose to let go of the strain. We can take a walk or do stretches, allowing our body to move again. We can wiggle, bounce, spin, wave our arms, roll our shoulders and our eyes — any motion we can think of to shake loose the tension. We can breathe deeply, throwing our arms out wide to inhale and curling into a ball when we exhale, so that our whole body breathes.

Then, standing very still, we will feel the tingle and pulse of life coursing through us. Feeling this tangible connection with the energy of the Tao, we relax and remember that this is where our hope is fulfilled. As our breath moves freely in our body, so our ancient, innate wisdom will carry us as life unfolds.

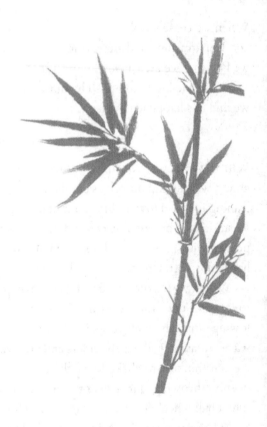

Letting Ourselves Be Carried

Since the Tao has given birth to all things
and fills all things,
it alone can care for all things
as a mother cares for precious children.

If we are called to render care,
we must watch and see
the subtle movements of the Tao.
We must move when it moves,
act when it acts,
and rest when it rests.
If our arms are to carry another,
we must let ourselves be carried.

THE EMOTIONAL AND PHYSICAL TURMOIL of caregiving seems all-encompassing. We can become so focused on providing care that we let go of everything that supports our own well-being. We begin to believe that we are on our own, that no one else can provide the care that we are providing. We see no other option but struggling on through to exhaustion.

From this perspective, we are unaware that all this is happening within a much broader context. There are others around us who would gladly care for us in this difficult time. Allowing them to do this, we open to the flow of compassionate care from the Tao, which may be expressed by the friend who really listens to us. It may be the flavor of homemade soup brought in by a neighbor. It may be the comfort of our bed when someone else is watching over our loved one. In all these small, important ways, we discover that we are indeed held in the embrace of mother Tao.

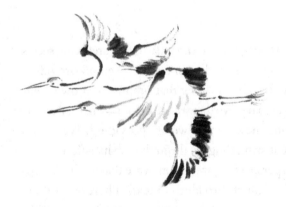

At Home within Ourselves

Restless energy keeps saying,
"Not this, something else."
It keeps us looking for an escape,
a return to something called "normal."

The Tao is never restless.
If we walk along its Way
we see the ever-changing sights
but do not lose ourselves in them.
We always remain at home within ourselves,
and our restless energy
settles of its own accord.

THAT URGENT FEELING that we must do something right away is the beginning of what we call a "suffering cycle." It begins with sensations in the body that may be tight, jittery, or bouncy. We label them "restless" and begin telling ourselves stories about what they mean. The more we believe that we must do something about being jittery, the more the tension builds. At the cycle's peak, we divert ourselves to break the stress. We will do anything to escape this restlessness.

When we catch this cycle building, we do have another choice. We can sit with all this unsettled energy. We can experience the physical sensations without attaching labels or meanings. When we do, we discover that the sensations will peak and then ebb away.

We do not need to make ourselves calm. Everything quiets down on its own. Over time, we find that it is just a jittery feeling, nothing more. If we let it, it will pass through.

No Fixed Rules

There are no fixed rules of caregiving
that will assure us of being right
instead of wrong.
Intuition must be our trusted guide,
though it may lead us
down unknown paths.
An open mind is our greatest asset,
using every circumstance for good
and turning every mistake into benefit.
A receptive heart is our refuge.
Giving and receiving care
become the same experience.
This is the great secret of caregiving.

THERE IS NO WAY TO KNOW another person's experience. Simply choosing what we think is best for another clouds our ability to discover what he knows he needs. One of the hardest experiences for caregivers is allowing the one in our care to try standing on legs that may not hold his weight. We are not to let him fall, but we need to let him try. This act of self-reliance is more important to him than safety.

What if there is nothing wrong with trying and nothing wrong with the sadness we share when he fails? Can we bring openness and compassion as we sit side by side on the floor? We are just two people, catching our breath. In a few minutes we will figure out together how we might get back to the chair.

The Oneness of All Things

Caregiving unites the opposing forces of life:
being active when necessary,
yet knowing the value of rest;
working to restore health,
yet accepting illness;
experiencing all emotions,
yet taking nothing personally;
honoring life,
yet accepting its transience;
seeing separate forms and functions,
yet knowing the Oneness of all things.

Caught in our conditioned mind
we try to separate the opposites,
having one without the other.
When we return to our Tao mind,
the opposites work together
for our highest good.

ALL OUR EXPERIENCES JOIN TOGETHER to make life rich, precious, and mysterious. The one who has never been ill or injured assumes she has mastered her body and that it will always behave as she expects it to. For her, serious illness or approaching death seems confusing and unfair. The body has betrayed her. There should be a way to regain control. Yet this physical form has been changing and shifting throughout her life, without her permission.

When we are a companion to another's dying, we find that we are witnessing life continue one breath at a time, until there is an exhale not followed by an inhale. It has been this way since birth, but now living takes on a new beauty and depth because we can foresee its end.

When life includes all the points on the continuum, it becomes full and vibrant. There is nothing outside the basic unity. Since all is held in this Oneness, there is nothing we have to cling to and nothing we need to push away.

No Separation

If we try to fix the situation,
we separate ourselves from it.
Separate from it,
we cease to understand it.
Not understanding it,
we try to control it.
Trying to control it,
we suffer.

If we become one with the situation,
we know exactly what to do.
Not holding ourselves separate,
we understand.
Understanding,
we accept the ebb and flow.
Accepting the ebb and flow,
we remain at peace.

IN OUR PRACTICE SIMPLE RITUALS help support us in being fully present in this moment. One of these is the series of bows we make as we enter the meditation hall. At the doorway, we pause and bow, with the silent reminder that we are letting go of everything past and future to come to this place with our full attention.

When we reach our cushion, we bow to it and commit to remaining here with our open awareness throughout this meditation time or class. Silently we repeat that we are willing to be here. Then we turn and bow to the hall and commit to remaining open to those who share this path with us. We are all held in acceptance and gratitude on this journey.

As we move into the room of the one in our care, we may want to carry similar silent reminders. We are willing to drop what we have been doing and our plans for later on. We are willing to be right here. In this way we find our place in what is emerging now.

[30]
Just This

Knowing what to do is not as important
as knowing when to stop doing it.
Resisting the way things are
keeps us trapped in a loop
of doing and striving.

If we believe our conditioned mind,
there is never a time when we can stop doing.
There is always more to do.

If we trust our Tao mind,
times to stop and rest appear like rainbows,
surprising us in the cloudy sky.
Pay attention to these times.

IT MAY BE A GLIMPSE OF THE MOON partnered with the morning star as we make an early cup of tea. It may be noticing the bare tree branches against the deep blue of the sky. It may be the tiny pause between the end of an exhale and the beginning of an inhale. Life is filled with gifts of rest and renewal. The activity that captivates our attention in this moment can quiet the incessant chatter of conditioned mind. At each moment, we can choose to focus on some simple bit of beauty or comfort in our surroundings.

For now there is the feeling of warm soapy water on our hands as we caress the bowl that held this evening's stew. Whatever we are doing, right this moment, can be a place of renewal and rest. All we need to do is sink into the gift of "just this."

Not Going to War

Despite popular slogans,
we are not battling diseases or misfortunes
when we act as caregivers.
To imagine our situation a battlefield
is to put ourselves at war with life.
We see enemies everywhere.
Even the one we care for
becomes someone to contend with.

We are bringing compassion,
not aggression.
We are sharing an experience,
not going to war.

OUR CULTURE HAS ELEVATED the image of fighting against illness and death. This image adds struggle, strain, and the fear of defeat to the challenges already inherent in illness or injury. It calls for heroic efforts from those who may be doing all they can just to make it through the day. In the end, the time comes to let go. This may consist of adjusting to reduced physical ability because the body has recovered as much as it can. It may be acknowledging that life is ebbing away and that no force of will can stop the process.

We stand as true companions to the ones we care for when we honor their experience. We listen when they tell us that it is time to stop struggling and rest. In this way we allow their days to be filled with tenderness, sadness, and gratitude rather than the efforts of battle and war.

Trust the Tao

Medical diagnoses and prognoses
create the illusion of predictability
and control.
Life's mysteries are too subtle
for prediction and control.

Medical knowledge may be helpful,
but it is not the substance of your caring.
Beneath the knowledge lies this truth:
All forms arise from the Tao,
live in the Tao,
and return to the Tao.

Use your knowledge,
but trust the Tao
for the arising, living, and returning.

THE DAY MAY COME WHEN YOU REALIZE that you are lost in measuring medications, learning how to change dressings, and managing various symptoms. Your focus has narrowed to one body part and then the next. You try to get all the new symptoms down on paper, hoping that someone can tell you what they mean and what will happen next.

When that day comes, broaden your vision to include the whole room. Notice the light coming through the window. Take in the color and texture of the blanket on the bed. Now let your gaze rest on the person in the bed. Take time to look in her eyes and to reconnect with her.

Here you will rediscover the ageless wisdom of the Tao that guides all living and dying. This broader perspective allows you to combine the medical information with your innate wisdom. You are here to bring tender care to this amazing human being.

[33]
Healing Ourselves

Understanding what another person feels
is helpful knowledge.
Knowing what we ourselves are feeling
is essential wisdom.
Easing another's pain
requires a certain kind of skill.
Easing our own suffering
requires true power.

Healing ourselves
is the greatest act of caregiving.

MUCH OF OUR SUFFERING stems from believing that we know what other people think and feel. We act on these assumptions, only to feel hurt and rejected when our words and actions are not welcome.

In our Tao mind, we take nothing personally and remain with our own experience. We cannot know what our care receivers are experiencing. Their attention moves from one physical sensation to another and from one internal story to the next. Their response is not about us, but a reflection of the inner work they are doing. Stepping back, we look at our own heart. What are we really experiencing? What are the fears and anxieties, the hopes and expectations that we carry right now? Can we focus compassion on our own heart where the turmoil exists?

Considering these questions, we reenter our direct experience. We do not need to understand what others are going through. Accepting our own inner dynamics, we find new balance and calm. We can wait, open and available, so we will be ready when they can share what they need.

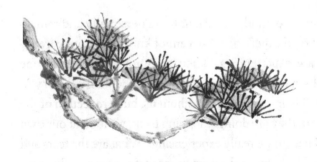

No Separate Self

The Tao does not think of itself as
"The Great Tao."
It does not think of itself at all;
thus it does not separate itself from us.
This is why it is called Great.

The more we think of ourselves,
the more we feel separate and
the more we suffer.
But trying not to think of ourselves
is to be constantly thinking of ourselves.
Our caring is at its best
when there is no thinking,
no separate self.

WE HAVE LEARNED TO BELIEVE that the endless stream of thoughts in our mind exists to help us distinguish "me" from "you." Their commentary provides information so each of us can know who "I" am. The "me" created by these thoughts becomes the star in countless internal dramas about how "I" am doing and what others think about "my" actions.

In truth, these are only thoughts. They have no form or substance. They mean nothing about our true nature. We practice letting go of thoughts as we notice them. Not clinging and not pushing them away, we find that they fade away from our lack of interest. Now there is nothing separating us from life or from those we share it with. Our attention rests on whatever is before us in this moment.

Life is more interesting than any story our mind can tell about it. Why would we allow anything to separate us from life?

When All Else Fails

We turn to the Way of the Tao
when other approaches fail.
If we had turned to this Way earlier
we would have suffered less,
but we keep trying to make things work.
Silence and gentle acceptance
do not appeal to our conditioned mind,
so we stick with noise
and empty promises,
which finally wear us out.

When we are worn out,
we turn to the Tao
and find a peace within all the changes
and an inexhaustible energy for our work.

OUR WHOLE LIVES OUR CONDITIONED MIND has worked to push us through our days. It insists that if we just tried harder, we could make life what we want it to be. It demands more effort to control both what happens and how we feel about what happens. In the midst of caring for someone in a health crisis, this pressure can feel unrelenting.

If we are fortunate, the time comes when our conditioned mind pushes us off an internal cliff. In utter despair, we give up trying to do the impossible. There may be sobbing and grief as we let go, but we fall into the grace of our true nature. The Way of the Tao opens up before us. It invites us to trust what runs deep within. Life will unfold in, around, and through us. It is not up to us to make things happen.

This is not helplessly giving up. It is stepping with courage into the reality of life. Within the flow of the Tao we find new confidence, peace, and joy. We are ready to sit still and wait to see where the journey will lead us.

Acceptance Sets Us Free

If we want a situation to change,
we must let it remain as it is.
If we want people to heal,
we must let them be ill.
If we want to be strong
we must let ourselves be weak.

Resistance keeps us stuck.
Acceptance sets us free.

WHEN WE ARE CONFRONTED WITH CIRCUMSTANCES that are not what we want them to be it is natural to push back against them. We want to change them, deny them, or make them go away. We communicate to the one in our care that she is not who we want her to be — someone who is whole, healthy, vigorous. We communicate to ourselves that we are not who we want to be — someone who is energetic, in control, and at ease with life. We can both end up discouraged and withdrawn.

When we notice this tension and yield, our experience is transformed. In accepting that this set of symptoms and these challenges are just what is happening in this moment, we find solid ground. When we acknowledge what it real, our vision clears. Now we can see what is possible, given the energy and strength we have today.

Does Itself

Caregiving may seem complicated
and difficult.
But for the Tao mind,
it is simple and easy.
It holds no tension in the body
or struggle in the mind.

Each thing comes according to its nature
and goes when the time is right.
If we resist the temptation to interfere,
the situation will find its way to peace.
When our mind is in the Tao,
caregiving simply does itself.

WHEN WE ASSUME THAT TAKING CHARGE is part of providing
care, we are caught in our conditioned desire for control. We
take on responsibility for what will happen and for how things
should be done. We can end up forcing our way forward, creating the resistance and fear we are here to ease.

One of our key tasks is to take the time to see what this
moment holds. The person in front of us will not be the same
as he was thirty minutes ago. The calm and confident one who
was ready for anything may have shifted to a worried child
who wants to withdraw. We need to take the time to see who
it is we are here to support.

Then we need to honor his lifetime by giving him choices
about how we go about the task at hand. Our way may be
efficient, but if it leaves him feeling out of control, he may

hesitate to ask the next time he needs help. Our best preparation for providing care is to enter gently and to bring our full awareness to this person as he is right now. When we do, we can work together as a trusting team to do whatever is needed with greater ease.

38

We Are Good

Not trying to be good,
we are free to truly care.
When we try to be good,
our caring loses power.
We work harder
and accomplish less.

Trying to be good
is a pale imitation of caring.
It blooms like a flower for a moment,
but it fades soon after blooming.
Our caregiving is the fruit at the center of life,
not the flower.
We don't have to try to be good.
We are good.

WE ALL HAVE A NATURAL DESIRE to express goodness. In childhood, this innate goodness became overlaid with definitions and meanings as we experienced the approval and disapproval of those around us. Many of us were taught that if we were not careful we would end up being "bad."

Whether we are working as caregiving professionals or serving members of our family, it is not unusual for us to feel the grip of this conditioning. If we are not aware of it, our work becomes much more difficult. We try hard to please and end up frustrated, discouraged, or rebellious when we don't get the response we expect.

Trusting our inherent goodness, we act naturally out of

our compassion and wisdom. There is no need to weigh and judge what we will do or how others react. We do not need to try to be good. Goodness came to us at our first breath.

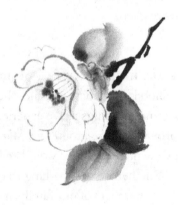

Humility

Despite our seeming maturity,
we know that we are little children,
utterly dependent on the Tao
and helpless without it.
So we care for others with humility.

We do not act as if we are virtuous
or possessors of a special power
but as if we know how fragile
and precious life is.
How can we help but be kind?

EVERY YEAR WE WATCH the cycle of living, dying, stillness, and rebirth in the turning of the seasons. The leaves of the fall trees blaze in glorious color. They gradually fade and then fall. When the gray of winter ebbs, the ends of the branches will show the tiny green fringe of new leaves budding. It is soothing to know that our lives are unfolding in this same ageless rhythm. Life is fragile and transient, and this makes it rich and vibrant.

Understanding this can add layers of wonder to our care-giving. Those in our care know that their hold on life and health is tentative. They become our guide, taking time to really taste a bite of cinnamon roll. They patiently watch the play of wind in the branches of a tree.

This fall, we know that we may never share another change in the seasons. There is one leaf left on the maple tree outside, and the rain is starting to fall. We grow still, sitting next to each other. Today we will just watch in case we get to see that last leaf float gently to the ground.

[40]
No Independent Existence

Everything in the universe is uniquely itself
yet is also part of everything else
and depends on everything else.

There is no independent existence.
In caring for another person,
we ourselves are cared for.

WE MAY THINK THAT PROVIDING CARE is all about giving to
someone else. We do things out of love for another person that
we would never attempt otherwise. Our willingness to be of
service overpowers our fear and uncertainty. We do what the
moment requires because of our commitment to be here for
those we love.

As the relationship unfolds, we discover more and more
what a gift our caregiving is to us. We hear the stories of a lifetime, imbued with the transparency of being told for the last
time. These tales reveal the wonder of this unique person,
who is the culmination of decades of experiences and eons of
memories.

Within ourselves we discover courage and strength, en-
durance and willingness, tenderness and compassion that we
have never experienced before. In the sharing of this journey
of caregiving, we have discovered more of who we are.

A Paradox

We are a paradox to ourselves.
Part of us is ready and willing,
and another part is sometimes willing
and sometimes wants to back away.
Yet another part wants to run
as far away as possible,
as quickly as possible.

The Tao contains within its nature
abundant paradoxes.
That which seems difficult to do
is actually the easiest.
That which seems dirty and soiled
is actually the purest.
The action that seems harsh
is actually the most compassionate.
That which seems our weakest moment
is actually our strongest.

AS WE START GIVING CARE, we may look ahead to some task we fear we won't be able to do. From a distance the task seems like a cliff edge. We know we can go that far, but beyond that it is too frightening, messy, uncomfortable, and unpredictable. We are afraid that we will fail at giving care.

As we keep going, we find that we reach that cliff without noticing. We are doing what naturally unfolds, and suddenly here is the task we had dreaded. Now that it is here, there is no question that we will be able to keep going. What appeared too difficult is now just what needs to be done. The willingness we need arises. We do our best with as much tenderness as possible. The direct experience is just one more step along the way. It was not a cliff after all.

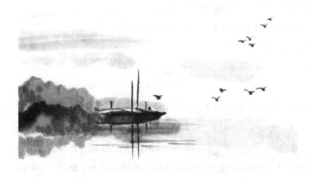

42

Yin and Yang

The energies of yin and yang combine
to hold the universe together,
but we dearly want to cling to one
and have the other go away.

We didn't want this to happen,
but it has.
We want to know what will happen tomorrow,
but we can't.
We can only stand here at the center
and watch and breathe.
We feel alone and helpless,
but we're not.
Life weaves itself around us,
making us a part of all that is.

FOR MANY OF US, there is one inside who tries very hard to change the outcome in painful situations. This one looks with tender innocence at the one in her care and wishes that he did not have to experience pain, sadness, confusion, or weakness. This one believes that if she tries hard enough, she can make things better. But she can't. There is no life without pain, no dying without discomfort, and no healing without struggle.

The result can be a wave of despair. When all our striving does not reverse an injury or cure an illness, there comes a moment of letting go. It may be with sorrow and tears, anger and frustration, or simple exhaustion — but it will come.

Then we are free. We no longer try to do the impossible. So we are available to do what we can. We will be a companion with a tender and open heart. That is the greatest gift we can give.

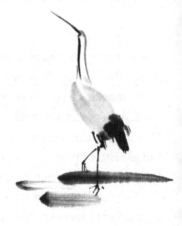

43

No Need to Bustle

Bustling about may seem helpful,
but stillness is the way of the Tao.
Filling the air with words may seem effective,
but silence is the way of the Tao.
We are taught to be busy,
and it is difficult to be still.
Most people choose a way of effort
and keep themselves unconscious
of the true nature of things.

Mindful actions
and a few words, gently spoken:
this is the movement of the Tao.

OFTEN WE DO NOT EVEN NOTICE that we are bustling in and out of another person's life. We have adopted an urgent pace, seeking to accomplish as much as possible in a limited time. We are going full speed in our speech and actions as we burst in on one whose day is unfolding very slowly. Instead, try this practice:

When you get to the door, pause before entering and take a deep breath. Drop the past and the future to be fully present with yourself in this moment.

Open the door slowly and enter as though you do not want to disturb the flow of what is happening in the room. Take time to sit down. Allow silence and listening to fill the emptiness.

When you speak, keep it simple. Ask a question, and allow the one you are caring for all the time he needs to give a response. Don't interrupt; just listen. This is a complex and wonderful human being, sharing with you the precious resources of his time and limited energy.

[44]
Nothing We Cannot Face

Peace awaits us in the midst of trouble.
Hidden in all that we don't want
lies that which we most desire.
We sometimes feel alone and helpless,
but our deepest needs are being met.
There is nothing we need to avoid,
and nothing we cannot face.

Amid the chaos we realize
that we are strong and capable.
Living in uncertainty, we discover
that we can be content.
Even in the midst of loss we find
that the whole world belongs to us.

WE ARE CAPABLE OF EXPERIENCING LIFE. It seems strange to
have to point that out, since our very existence proves that we
have been able to survive everything we have already encountered. But we often act as though we were not designed for
the complex blend of thoughts, emotions, and sensations that
is life. We believe that life is too painful and confusing for us.

When we drop this belief, everything opens up. This
does not mean that it will all be comfortable and easy. It
means that in the depth of our despair and helplessness, we find
that we are strong enough to take the next step. In the midst
of chaos and confusion, we can grow still, breathe, and wait
to see what is next.

As we face the most difficult challenges, we find that we
were created to experience life in all its intensity.

What Is Given

We are not trying to make things perfect,
nor are we trying to fill the hours with activity.
We are merely taking what is given,
nothing more.
We are working with what is
and adding nothing else.
We may feel inefficient, hesitant, and lost.
But these very qualities
bring us softness, gentleness,
and the ability to walk in the dark
without falling.

OUR CONDITIONED MIND loves to add endless commentary and opinion to every experience. Thoughts lead to meanings, and meanings lead to stories. We are told what has to happen and what must not happen. Very quickly we lose the direct experience of life in the confusion as we react to things that have never happened.

Being present in the moment, we return to "what is given." Life is perfect as it is. This moment between these two people has never happened since before the stars were born. There is no way we can know what it means and no way we can add anything to it.

When we drop all the rest and remain with "what is given," we will be present in this moment with compassion and gentleness. This is how we let in all the richness of life.

[46]

Let Thoughts Settle

When we are aware of the Tao
our work is simple and helpful.
When we lose sight of the Tao,
our work becomes complicated by fear.
Our helpfulness disappears,
and we resist each change that comes.

Return to your breath,
and let your thoughts settle for a moment.
You will rediscover the willingness waiting
at the center of your heart.

IT TAKES PRACTICE to let our awareness remain in the Tao. We long for it to be simple and natural, but for too many years our mind has wandered far and wide, finding suffering and fear. We must choose to return to our own heart and become familiar again with the ancient, innate wisdom within us.

We discover that tension in the body, urgency to take action, and resistance to what is happening are all signals that we are caught in conditioned mind. When we notice these things, we return to the physical sensation of the breath. It brings us back into our body and the direct experience of this moment.

When we trust again in our own heart, we discover the gracious unfolding of the Tao. There is nothing to figure out. Fear yields to a curiosity about what will happen next.

That Which Is Within

We may feel cooped up by our caregiving,
doomed to watch the world go by
outside our window.
Yet we are given a window
that opens on the heart —
a vista few people ever see.

We don't travel to faraway places,
yet knowledge, understanding, and wisdom
come to us right where we are.
It is not what is outside that satisfies,
but that which is within.

THERE IS NO WAY TO DESCRIBE THE VIVIDNESS of life that un-folds between caregiver and care receiver. There is no clearer view of our heart and mind. All our beliefs, hopes, and fears — even those we felt we had put to rest long ago — emerge with new intensity. We feel tension, fear, and uncertainty one moment and a breaking through into peace and confidence the next. We find that compassion is not a soft, delicate thing but that which brings clarity and courage.

We see total vulnerability in the one we are caring for. The tenderness, wisdom, and courage of her heart become visible as she struggles to control the flow of life and health. Here in this room, we discover more about ourselves and each other than many decades have revealed before. What a sweet, amaz-ing vista we are given as caregivers.

[48]

No Assumptions

The Tao allows us
to hold assumptions lightly.
Each day we assume less about
what should happen,
what will happen,
what will not happen,
and what it all means,
until we are finally free of all assumptions
and can do our work with ease.

ASSUMPTIONS ARE BELIEFS we have about the future based on our experiences of the past. They fail to acknowledge the unique nature of every human experience. These people and circumstances have not come together in this way since before the beginning of beginningless time. The only honest response to the question of what the day will hold is "I don't know."

These words, spoken with gentle openness, acknowledge the fluid nature of life. "I don't know" can invite us to remain open to what is happening right now. If it is a moment of strength and health, we can celebrate together without seeking added signs of recovery. If it is one of weakness and pain, we can endure it without adding fears about the future. We do not know what is ahead. We do not need to know. We are committed to traveling this road together, no matter what happens.

Hearts Open to All

When our hearts are open to all,
our caregiving is light and easy.
We give care to the grateful person
who deeply appreciates our effort.
We give care to the ungrateful curmudgeon
who reviles us and resents us as intrusive

Since our actions need no reward,
those who oppose us
and those who welcome us
are equally seen as friends.

TRUE CAREGIVING EMERGES from deep within our being and is not affected by the response of others. Our well-being is not influenced by either gratitude or rejection as they appear throughout our day.

Our care receivers are therefore free to express all the frustration, anger, and fear that are part of being ill or injured. They do not need to protect us from their foul moods, because we do not take them personally. Their words and actions mean nothing about who we are. They also mean nothing about who they are.

Letting go of all this, we emerge into the full power of our being. Living from our center, connected to the grace of our heart, there is no question about why we are here or if we will choose to provide care. We do this because it expresses our true nature. We would not miss this opportunity to bring compassion to ourselves and others.

Gateway to Freedom

Death lurks in the background
of everything we do.
For some
it is a fearful thing
to be avoided and pushed aside.
For others
it is an obsession
that crowds out the joy of living.

For a follower of the Tao
it is the gateway to freedom.
It releases us from all resistances,
all evasions,
and all illusions.
It helps us to truly live.

WE RECEIVE A GIFT FROM THE INTENSITY of knowing that these are the last weeks of life. The narrowing of life's tasks and the softening of our thoughts with weariness produce a unique broad awareness.

Meals become a few bites of a favorite food, with tastes and textures savored with great pleasure. The caregiver, watching the licking of lips, and the eyes closed to focus on the flavors, is reminded of the sweetness of life.

The subtle warmth of a hand and the texture of the wrinkled lines of an aging face are amazing. The giggles and the grunts, the sighs and the moans punctuated with the varied rhythm of breathing form a song of life.

And then there are the colors. The pale baby pink of a bath towel or the emerald green of the dish soap captures our attention. Even the layers of silvers and charcoals in the winter sky draw us into a comforting embrace. We get to experience the whole palette of life's intense feelings and sensations. When we are open to it all, it holds a beauty and richness that we will never forget.

51

We Truly Want To

The Tao gives birth to all things
but does not claim to own them.
All beings honor the Tao,
not because they are supposed to
but because they truly want to.

We do not take on caregiving
because we are supposed to.
Beneath the resistance and resentment,
under the fear and frustration,
is something big and spacious,
welcoming and generous.

We are doing this
because we truly want to.

MANY OF US ARE CHOSEN BY CIRCUMSTANCES to provide care for our parents, siblings, or grown children. If our earlier relationships were fraught with tension and the sense that we were never doing things "right," caregiving may hold the added challenge of these memories. We may even fall into the same patterns of interacting that made the relationship uncomfortable when we were young.

This becomes an opportunity to question all the old, hurtful, conditioned messages that emerge as we provide care. It is not always a comfortable process, but it can lead to liberation and freedom that will serve us the rest of our lives. What if the happiness or unhappiness of those in our care has never been about us? What if we have no idea what they feel about their life? What if each one of us is good enough, just as we are?

As the grip of conditioned mind eases, we may discover that there is one within us who is simply compassionate, caring, and generous in spirit. We find we are here because we want to be.

[52]
Ordinary Things

Finding the Tao,
we find our own true self.
When we stop a moment
and realize who we really are,
we begin to work intuitively,
without excess thought and drama.
We are often quiet
and less prone to distracting ourselves
with excess chatter.
We notice all the small
and ordinary things
that grace our lives.
We respond to what is
instead of to what we think
should be.

AS WE PROVIDE CARE FOR SOMEONE who is dying, we find that life gradually becoming simpler. As her energy ebbs, she no longer goes into the kitchen. Soon it is enough to move from the bed to the table. Eventually, all of life is happening within her bedroom. The most basic tasks of eating, sleeping, and providing personal care and gentle conversation fill the days and nights. We are both invited to let go of everything else.

When all the chatter and drama fade away, we find ourselves enjoying the simple treasures around us. There is the taste of tea and the gentle familiar curve of the cup that holds it. We are soothed by the fresh, green scent after a rain. We take time to carefully arrange the flowers in a vase, to honor the color and beauty they add to the bedside. Living in this quieter way, we sink into the peace of our own heart. We need very little to bring us joy.

53

Simple Action

Caregiving can be simple,
but we often make it complicated
by following our mind
down many futile paths.

Our conditioned mind promises relief
by suggesting one distraction,
and then another.
It presents a long list of things
we could be doing
instead of this.
So we eat and drink and shop,
yet do not find the promised relief.

Relief can only come
when we return to the simple action
offered to us in the present moment.

WE HAVE SPENT DECADES CREATING our unique list of distractions to help us escape unwanted sensations and moods. For many of us this has worked fairly well in most situations, so we have never gained confidence in our ability to stay with what we are feeling.

Caregiving may be one of the most uncomfortable, uncertain, and important things we have ever done. There seems to be no rest. Even when we are away from the one in our care, the list keeps rattling on in our head about the things we need to figure out and what we need to try next. So it is natural that we search for something to take our mind off all this distress.

True relief is right in front of us. It is the task that we are doing in this moment. We allow ourselves to be drawn in by the sights, sounds, textures, and movements. When we bring our full attention to just this one action, the situation no longer feels overwhelming. We do not need to escape. We are fine being here, one moment at a time.

Life Is Transformed

As we embrace the Tao,
our life becomes transformed.
Everyone around us feels the difference
and becomes more confident
amid the many issues
and concerns.

Nothing escapes our notice,
and we fully experience every moment.
Our caregiving transforms itself
into a time of wonder
and adventure.

How do we embrace the Tao?
By holding ourselves with great tenderness.

OUR CONDITIONED MIND sees self-discipline and effort as the way to transformation. After years of trying, we find that force of will and obedience to rules do not change our basic approach to life. The Tao mind knows that the human heart is opened through tenderness. Compassion empowers and guides our life. It touches us first and then moves outward to enfold each person and every moment of life.

When we return to the guidance of our own heart, compassion sustains our caregiving. The one in our care can relax into its gentle embrace, finding both strength and safety within it. It is this innate tenderness that fuels our willingness to move through the most difficult times. The compassion we need to sustain us will continue to well up from within our own heart.

Work without Resistance

In harmony with the moment,
we work all day.
We remain focused on our tasks
and never grow tired.

If we live within the moment,
neither our body
nor our mind resists.
Thus neither one exhausts itself.
Thoughts come and go.
Tasks come and go.
We remain as vital as a child at play.

IT IS AMAZING HOW MUCH ENERGY is drained from our life by the mental chatter that convinces us that this is not what we want to be doing. In fact, this resistance may torment us day and night with thoughts about how draining caregiving is and how unwelcome it is in our life. Listening to this endless loop of stories, we feel tense and tired, and no wonder.

When we see through the mental chatter, we can relax and regain our natural flexibility. Caregiving becomes a series of simple tasks that invite us to use one skill and then another. We soften as we find we can do each thing as it arises. We then let it go as the next task appears.

The mental chatter will continue. The secret is that when we stop believing its stories, this prattle no longer drains us. Life is a natural unfolding of experiences within the vast context of compassion. Here we can give and receive, work and rest.

Anonymous

The more we ruminate
and talk about our situation,
the less we really understand it.
The more we merely experience it,
the less we ruminate,
the less we talk,
and the more we understand.

It is best to let our thoughts
fade into a comfortable silence,
to listen,
to watch patiently,
to breathe fully,
to move mindfully,
and to remain quietly unnoticed
and anonymous like the Tao.

OUR CONDITIONED MIND is full of talking and ruminating, which serve drama rather than life. They take us away from what is actually happening to gather various opinions and comments from those around us. The story ends up being about us and how we appear to the outside world.

When we free ourselves of this dynamic, we can sink back into our direct experience. Bringing all our attention to this moment, we open to those before us. We discover that they are far more than a series of symptoms and care needs. We listen as they take on the depth and interest of the decades they have lived. The focus returns to these precious days. In silence we now enjoy being the witness to another person's life.

Not-Knowing

A plan of care may be helpful,
but the Tao cares without a plan.
The more we try to manage events,
the more they will surprise us.
In fact, the harder we try,
the more we fall short.
The more we control,
the less predictable we find things.

When we stop managing events,
events manage themselves.
When we stop trying to change things,
we find they change themselves.
No longer needing to know
what will happen next,
we find that life lives itself.
Not-knowing,
though frightening,
is true wisdom.

OFTEN WE ARE TEMPTED to focus our attention entirely on the tasks of managing care. Doing so gives us something tangible to do and keeps our minds occupied with goals. It is one of the ways we grasp for control. Life, however, refuses to be managed or predicted. The moment we are certain about what this day will hold, something new happens.

Our priority was to change a bandage, but instead we find

ourselves playing hide-and-seek with a favorite pair of gloves. It is okay to be surprised by life. Those things that truly need to be done will find their way into the day. For now we are looking under the dresser and in the pockets of every coat for that glove.

58

Holding Lightly

Hold all ideas
of what is good
and what is bad lightly.
What we want
and what we fear
are mixed together
in all events.

We have opinions and desires
but do not impose them on others.
We do not compound another's pain
by mixing it with our own.

We never truly know
what good can come
from what we call misfortune,
or what pain can arise
from what at first seemed fortunate.

WE EACH HAVE THEORIES about how living and dying should
unfold. Yet when we are the companion on the journey of
those in our care, we need to let go of these opinions. It is not
our place to add our hopes and fears to all they carry within
them. Released from these images, we can enjoy the unique
quality of these individuals' process of healing or declining.
Their response to each event can reveal new possibilities to us.

What we dread, they accept with ease. The change that

seems trivial to us challenges their sense of identity and freedom. We are deeply moved by their courage and peace, as well as their apprehension and struggle.

When our caregiving task is over, we become attuned to what we would have missed if we had not been invited to share these days.

Leave Yourself Room

The Tao always leaves room
for responding to any shift of direction.
It takes care of things as a mother
gently nurturing an infant,
letting her child rest
and eat
and play
in rhythm with nature.

Be moderate in your approach
to the unfolding of your day.
Avoid overzealous activity,
excessive self-criticism,
and ambitious goals.
Leave yourself room.

IN OUR CULTURE WE ARE OFTEN PRESSURED by hours on the clock and blocks on a calendar. Life is measured in hours and days, in care goals completed and visits made. If we nervously scan our watches or fidget with the passing minutes, we miss many moments of living.

Returning to Tao mind, we relax. We find ourselves shifting and changing with the rhythms of the day. We are with someone who no longer rises and rests according to a schedule. Meals and snacks are eaten when the tastes seem welcome and the stomach receptive. Today each conversation and every task will take as long as it takes. We abide in the calm awareness that there is nothing that has to be done that will not find its own way into the day. We trust in the flow of the Tao.

No Need for Force

Approach each day as if
you were frying a small fish.
If you poke it and stir it,
you will ruin it.
Don't force things,
don't hurry needlessly.
Hurry and force
are the result of inner fears
that arise from our conditioned habits
of worry and mistrust.

As we walk this path
we learn to trust
both ourselves
and those in our care.
The thought that used to cause us worry
now simply becomes
"just another thought."

SOME DAYS WE SEE EVERYTHING through the filters of our conditioned mind. We see only challenges, difficulties, and things that need to be done. In a single breath we can let go. Our caregiving is not any of these things. Rather, we are in a relationship with a fascinating human being.

Letting our focus rest gently on the day, we find unexpected gifts bubbling up. As we go about caring for others, they share stories no one else has ever heard. They teach us that brushing one's teeth and taking a shower can require our full attention to each detail of the process. They share the new trick they have learned in working around their weakness or pain.

If we are quiet and patient, we will see that this moment holds the culmination of a lifetime of laughter and tears, insights and foolishness. Imagine what we would have missed if we had hurried them through the day.

Receptive and Still

The Tao is like a valley.
It remains low
so all things may flow into it.
It serves everything that exists.

Those who need care
feel vulnerable and dependent.
The more dependent they feel,
the more humble we must be.
If we remain receptive and still,
not hiding our own vulnerable feelings
behind a role of power and authority,
we become a fertile valley.
Now we can provide
whatever nurturing is required.

WE ARE BY NATURE OPENHEARTED AND COMPASSIONATE.
Our conditioned mind seeks to convince us that it is too
painful to be vulnerable. It is a myth that we must appear
strong and unmoved by another person's struggle. Within our
hearts we feel tenderness, sadness, longing, courage, and sorrow. It is compassion that allows all of life's intensity to flow
through.

As we reclaim our true nature, we choose to be vulnerable. We trust our ability to feel everything that arises and the
freedom to let it show in our eyes. The one in our care is en-
folded in this same trust. Neither of us needs to hide or endure
pain, fear, or anger alone. The Tao nurtures both of us through
it all.

Part of Each Other

The Tao is a source of peace
for those who need care
and a refuge
for those who give it.
Within the Tao we are not two beings,
forever separate and apart.
We are part of each other
in a manner we cannot truly fathom.
But in the circumstances
that have brought us together,
we feel and know
that this is true.

We honor ourselves
by caring for others.
We honor others
by caring for ourselves.

A MYSTERIOUS, TRANSFORMING POWER resides in the relationship of giving and receiving care. We think we are giving care for the sake of the other, but the experience will change our lives. While we might have thought that we were not ready for this role, the wisdom of the Tao has brought us to it.

The caregiving experience begins as something that may seem very simple, but it draws all our deepest beliefs and desires into plain view. It can bring intensity to so many aspects of our life that we usually pull back and hide from. But now there is this other person, and we know in our hearts that we will see this through to honor him or her.

The ancient, inherent wisdom that has always been within us emerges to help us trust in the refuge of the Tao. This creates the safety we need to allow fear and sorrow, laughter and tears to shake us free from a lifetime of conditioning. We honor each other in the way we share this path, becoming more and more visible to each other along the way.

63

Free of Stories

Caring for another person
seems an awesome task,
yet we do it without effort.
Small events of the day
are fascinating to us.
Difficult moments reveal to us
our own authentic kindness.
Complicated tasks are seen
as a series of simple steps.
Fatigue is just a tired feeling,
free of stories and dramatic meaning.

In the midst of all this work,
we find that many mental habits
that used to cause us suffering
have simply disappeared.

PART OF BEING IN THE TAO as a caregiver is letting go of the dramas of the mind so that life can flow through. We recognize that our fatigue comes from doing a good day's work and from learning the skills of providing care that sometimes change with each passing hour.

Like small children we are completely captivated by each experience as it unfolds. We move from one caring task to the next, interested in how this body works and in the personality of the one in our care. In each moment we can allow ourselves to be in a creative dance as we try new things and discard options that no longer serve.

At the end of the day, we fall into a heap. There is nothing wrong with feeling tired. We let every muscle relax and every thought dissolve. There is nothing more to do, and no stories to tell about the day.

64

Stillness Shows the Way

Sitting still is hard to do.
We want to do something,
somehow change things
and help someone.
But the journey may be long,
and we cannot see
where the path is leading.

Great patience is required.
Stillness shows the way.
In the stillness we plant the seed
from which the tree may grow.
We stop and notice the only essential step
in the journey of a thousand miles —
the next one.

WHEN A HEALTH CRISIS INITIALLY OCCURS, we easily shift into a sprint to do everything we can. We may put our own routines on hold to sit at a hospital bedside or to travel across country to be with someone who is desperately hurt or ill.

When that initial urgent stir begins to ebb, we find that we need to shift to a long, slow, easy lope. There are hours of sitting and waiting to see what will happen. In the uncertainty we develop an internal stillness. We find ourselves living one moment at a time. There is no hurry and no need to foresee what lies ahead. The scenarios of recovering full health or letting go of life will unfold in their own time.

When we feel that sense of urgency arising, we return to

our breath. Placing a hand on our belly, we can feel its rising and falling. We enter the rhythm of the breath as it enters the body, fills the body, and then leaves the body. We will sit here, following the breath and waiting. There is nothing else we have to do.

65

No Experts

The great heroes on this path
are unknown and unsung.
Throughout the ages they have worked
with humble simplicity,
merely one person helping another
through the ordinary trials of life.

Looking to experts
will make us lose our way.
The power of the Tao
comes from within each person's heart.
We merely help reveal this power
to those for whom we care.
We may help them do things
they cannot do themselves,
but the power within them
remains their true caregiver.

WE MAY LONG FOR AN EXPERT TO APPEAR and do everything for us, to protect us from facing things we have never tried before. We want to escape the uncertainty and tension of unfamiliar tasks. Yet we develop some of our most useful skills when we have no other choice. We trust that what we may lack in expertise we will make up for with our deep intention to be kind and tender.

The first time we change a bandage or help someone find a comfortable position in bed we feel slow and awkward. But in taking our time, we notice the little things that might make it easier the next time. In all this those in our care are the experts about their own minds and bodies. Even in this unknown territory they know how to proceed.

When the moment comes, we will bring patience and compassion for each other. We bring our willingness to try, and those we care for bring their gratitude that there is someone to help do what they cannot. Together we make the way ahead a little easier.

Remain Behind

When caring for others,
remain behind them.
Help them,
but do not control them.
Serve them,
but do not manipulate them.
Attend them,
but do not diminish them.

The river of the Tao
runs through them.
Stay out of the way,
and let that river do its work.

ONE DAY WE MAY NOTICE that an unconscious shift has happened between us and the one in our care. We had been ready to assist with the tasks he chose for the day. Now we take over and decide that it would be easier if we just did those things for him. We notice the subtle way we talk him out of doing something that is important to him because we are not sure it is worth the energy and effort.

When we notice this shift, we can return to the heart of our caregiving. We can step back and take a long, deep breath. We can let our focus rest on this man who has lived as an independent adult for decades and has overcome many obstacles. He is capable of guiding his care. Time and energy are a small price to pay to honor this unique expression of the Tao as he moves through these difficult days.

Ordinary Caregiving

Some would call it heroic,
a path for extraordinary people.
But caregiving is really very ordinary.
It is just the Tao expressing itself
in everyday events.

Three virtues
help us along the way:
compassion, simplicity, and patience.
When we have compassion,
we find that fear is gone
and that tenderness replaces toughness.
When we have simplicity,
we find that the need for control is gone
and that generosity takes its place.
When we have patience,
we no longer strive and strain.
Peace becomes our natural experience.

BE VERY WARY OF THE CONDITIONED VOICE that wants to call caregiving heroic and to describe our work as arduous. While this voice may sound as if it is offering encouragement, it may well be driving us to "strive hard" and to take this on as a "valiant effort." Suddenly, what we have enjoyed as daily life with a loved one or as a chosen profession that allows us to care for others becomes something requiring superhuman strength.

Let go of all that. It is the way caregiving weaves us into the most common human experiences that fills it with honor

and reward. From the beginning of time, caring for one another has been an expression of our natural connection.

It is all right to enjoy this time and to find playfulness in
the midst of it. Caregiving gives us permission to experience
tenderness and to celebrate the quiet moments of life.

No Pretense

Circumstances may be painful,
but we do not fight to overcome them,
nor do we fight to overcome ourselves.

When we feel weak,
we do not pretend that we feel strong.
Thus our weakness helps us to understand ourselves
and keeps us tender and compassionate.
When we feel strong
we act with calm effectiveness.
Thus our strength truly benefits others.
Both our weakness and our strength
are used for helpful purpose.

CAREGIVING MAY INVITE US TO SPEND OUR ENERGY, risking
both fatigue and weakness. We might not even notice this fatigue building, because we keep doing the next thing, adjusting anew to the lack of a regular schedule.

When we are physically and mentally drained, we can accept this as part of the caregiving experience. While we continue our work, it helps to acknowledge that this is just how we feel today and that we will simply do what we can.

We also learn to rest when we have the opportunity. This includes dismissing the mental inventory that wants to captivate us at 2:00 AM. Even as we have learned to be fully present while providing care, we practice being fully present with ourselves in our times away.

When it is time to sleep, we return to the breath and the

sensation of the bed supporting our weight. We allow every muscle to relax, and we let vigilance melt away. Then, as our energy naturally returns, we reenter our caregiving with clarity and gentleness. The same awareness that supported our rest is now available for our day's work. We enter fully into the next step along the way, giving ourselves over to what is ours to do.

69

A Part of All That Happens

These circumstances did not arise
to purposefully make us suffer.
They are not a plot
to keep us in a constant struggle,
to get us to wrest some peace from turmoil,
and finally triumph over our cruel fate.

Our peace comes when we let go
and see the whole of life
instead of the tiny, separate parts.
Our triumph arrives when we become
a part of all that happens
rather than apart from it.

LIFE IS NOT SOME EXTERNAL FORCE trying to teach us lessons, make us stronger, or humble us. It is not something outside us, throwing us challenges and tests to see how we react.

This feeling of separation comes from creating our own imaginary walls. These walls claim to protect us from the aspects of life that are too painful or uncertain for us. Instead, they keep us feeling cut off from our true capacity for living.

The caregiving experience may be uncomfortable, since it asks for those dividing walls to come down. Yet as they do, we discover that we have an inner strength we did not recognize. We are more willing to take full responsibility for our own experience than ever before.

We even recognize our connection to the peace, power,

and eternal guidance of the Tao. They reside within our heart and flow freely as we recognize that all of life is available to us. We have all we need.

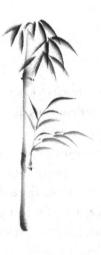

70

As Effortless as Breathing

In conditioned mind
caregiving seems difficult,
full of struggle and resentment.
In Tao mind,
it is as natural
and effortless as breathing.

Caring for others
with conditioned mind
will bring exhaustion
to ourselves and to them.

But caring that arises from the Tao
is simple, effortless, and natural.
It will bring freedom and peace
to everyone involved.

THERE IS A KIND OF GRACE in becoming captivated by the present-moment tasks of providing care for one you love. This is not the narrow focus of conditioned mind trying to drive you from morning to night. It is the broad, open awareness that this is simply what you are doing today.

It doesn't matter if the internal negative stories prattle on. When your focus rests gently on what you are doing, those voices take on a cloudlike quality — they have no power and cannot hold your attention.

People around you try to compliment you on the

wonderful thing you are doing. But you know that this is not about trying to be a good caregiver. There is no effort in being here. It is natural to travel this path of caring together.

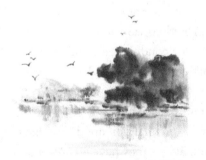

An Ever-Growing Awe

There is no real difference
between caregiver
and care receiver.
We are each of us in awe,
and sometimes very frightened,
of the mystery of life.

Together we learn to trust
and gradually replace the fear
with an ever-growing awe.

WE CAN GET INTO A KIND OF DANCE with our care receivers
in which we both put on a brave face. We both work to hide
the fear that arises as we discover how much of life is beyond
our control.

There are the half-smiles and the furrowed brows. There
are words of encouragement that are more for the speaker's
benefit than the listener's. We repeat to each other that we are
both doing fine. Then one of us breaks free to give a tremen-
dous gift. The words are spoken: "I think we both need to ad-
mit that we are scared."

In that moment we are set free. All the distance created by
pretending falls away. We no longer focus on the fear, but look
into each other's eyes. Yes, we are both afraid. Yes, we are both
okay in our fear. Now we can move forward in spite of the
fear, because its power is diminished by our mutual acceptance
and love.

Only the Tao

Without reverence for the Tao
we become overwhelmed by pain and loss
and our experience is controlled by fear.
With reverence we are not afraid.
We do not constrict our life
by spinning scary stories.
We cherish others as ourselves
and ourselves as others.
In our mind there is no "self"
and "other."
There is only the Tao
manifesting itself in ever-changing,
limitless forms.

WE ARE NOT MERELY INDIVIDUALS bouncing life back and forth between us. The caregiving process cannot be segmented into one giving and one receiving, one acting and the other responding. We are all expressions of one process of life unfolding. Our true nature is to live in harmony with all of life.

Our wisdom and clarity do not emerge in isolation but are born in the space we share with others. In our interaction, new insights become visible, and we discover who we are in new ways.

Within this caregiving relationship something new is coming into being in the thoughts, actions, and feelings that emerge. Our experience of life grows and changes each moment in response to what we both bring to it.

The awe and wonder inherent in this process leave little

room for fear. The pain and loss well up and flow into greater tenderness. Laughter and love grow to add to the joy of the days ahead. Everything we are finds expression in this care-giving relationship. Each interaction brings a new taste of how the Tao manifests itself in limitless ways.

73

Help or Harm?

How can we ever know
if we are truly being helpful?
We have no grand plan
for making everything better.
We can't be sure that what we do
brings help
or harm.
We don't know if help
will turn to harm,
or if harm will turn to help.

Without a plan,
and without knowing,
we remain patient
and attentive to the moment.
We do the best we can.

OFTEN AS CAREGIVERS we find that our attempts to bring comfort and to avoid pain do not work. Repositioning someone in bed causes discomfort but prevents the ache of muscles that have been in one position for too long. Physical care is absolutely necessary, and yet often it results in moans and grimaces.

If we allow our conditioned mind to pull us into a debate about harm and help, we will likely hurry through the task. Trying to avoid our own discomfort in this moment, we pull, push, and force our way through the care that must be given. We block the reaction of this dear person in our care so that we can convince ourselves that we know what has to be done.

In these times we can choose to trust our innate desire to provide tender care. When we do, the calm, stable point of reference within will allow us to take our time. We can stay present to those receiving our care and acknowledge their pain and struggle.

In this way, pain has not been turned to suffering: not for them, and not for us.

74

Nothing Left to Fear

All things are transient,
and change is the constant of the Tao.
Clinging causes pain,
but letting go seems so hard.

We know the final change is death
for our loved ones
and for ourselves.
Fear of this final change
brings fear of all changes.
No wonder we resist
and cling with such tenacity.
But when we see
that even death, which
we call "the final change"
may itself be changed in turn,
our life gives way to freedom
and there is nothing left to fear.

WE ALL KNOW INTELLECTUALLY that the final outcome of living is dying. Yet so much fear surrounds the unknown and uncontrollable nature of death that our minds keep us from seeing that our loved one is dying.

We can see all the signs and symptoms. We have gotten into the pattern of taking one change and then the next in stride. We make countless adjustments to the amount and kind of care we give. Still, death remains veiled from our sight.

Fear keeps awareness just out of reach, and we suffer without knowing why.

Then one day the illusion shatters. It becomes real that the one we love is dying. There are tears and sorrow but also relief and freedom. We can stop trying to change the outcome. Life is ending, as it has for all beings throughout time. There is nothing left to fear.

Learn from Them

It is not necessary to intrude,
nor do we have to meddle.
People can be trusted with their lives.
Even when we may feed them,
bathe them,
and clothe them,
we do not lead their lives for them.
They lead their lives themselves.

In everything we do
we leave a space for them.
They alone know what to do,
how to live,
when to hold on,
when to struggle,
and when to let go.

REGARDLESS OF OUR ROLE or our relationship to those in our care, we must never lose sight of their humanity and individuality. As they decline in physical strength and mental clarity, it is even more important for us to guard their dignity.

We are here to listen, to attend to them, and to see them as clearly as we can. We are here to honor who they have always been: an amazing expression of the Tao.

The process of aging and dying is the culmination of decades of living. They bring their unique insights and accumulated life experiences to the unfamiliar tasks of this time. Allowing them to direct our actions as much as possible, we will continue to learn from them, right up through their last breath.

Soft and Supple

Whatever we do
we do not stiffen
and let the situation make us rigid.

We remain soft and supple
like the branches of a sapling.
Whatever storms may come,
our spirit stays flexible.
Not attached to outcome,
we are not uprooted by the gales.

Rooted, but not rigid,
we move naturally in the winds of change,
bending but never broken.

PROVIDING CARE can be like being caught out in a storm. Our first instinct is to escape this untamed situation, measuring our strength by our ability to remain unswayed by its power. When we are alienated from our own hearts, we find it painful to witness another person's struggle.

When we open to our hearts, we can welcome the whole experience in a new way. The storm holds not only threat but also energy and excitement. Our responses become more natural as we let ourselves be moved by the moment.

When tears come, they are free to pour forth in sobs. When laughter bubbles up, we find that we giggle together over the silliest things. Living with flexibility, accepting all that comes our way, we find we can take in all the power and wonder of life.

We weather this storm, not by brute strength, but by remaining rooted in the Tao and yielding to the natural flow of life.

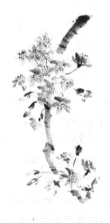

77

The Joy of Tender Caring

A bow holds tension in perfect balance:
Bend . . . release!
The arrow flies true to its target.
Too much tension,
the bow snaps.
Too little tension,
the arrow falls short.

Caregiving holds the same balance:
Effort . . . ease.
Too much effort,
we break beneath the strain.
Too much ease,
we lose the satisfaction of compassion
and the joy of tender caring.

THE TAO MIND RECOGNIZES THE SUBTLETIES of blending effort with ease and attentiveness with trust. This balance gives us the freedom to stay with our own experience rather than becoming overprotective of the one in our care.

We are walking next to the one we are caring for. We are watching for any hint that he is off balance so that we can quickly reach in and prevent a fall. The difficulty is that our heightened vigilance only makes both of us tense and rigid. We focus on avoiding a fall instead of walking alongside a man.

By placing a hand on the small of his back, we bring our attention back to our experience. We experience subtle shifts in the palm of our hand. We learn the feel of his gait and trust that if there is a sudden change, we will notice.

We are present, alert, and relaxed. We are both looking and moving in the same direction, sharing the experience of getting some fresh air.

78

Fluid and Flowing

The softness of water is deceiving.
Fluid and flowing,
it adapts to any situation.
Yet rocks and mountains
dissolve in its presence.

Opening ourselves to another person
is like releasing a river of compassion.
The gentle heart has the power
of a rushing stream.
In the presence of another's need,
our spirit remains supple and fluid.
Our flexible nature dissolves
the rigid structures of fear.

IT IS NOT ROCK-SOLID STABILITY or consistent daily routines that provide the strength we need to provide care. In fact, when we are captivated by maintaining these structures, we can miss many opportunities.

Water's flow may seem a vague and inefficient image for giving care. Yet it invites us to see clearly what is before us and to understand how to move around the obstacles blocking our way.

It may be that our care receivers are focused on processing the experiences of their life and what their physical condition means about who they are. Their priority is different from ours when we come into their room. Seeing this, we listen to them as they tell us what they need, rather than pushing forward with a plan of care.

Each day their needs for food and rest, activity and companionship, inward reflection and outward involvement will present themselves in new ways. The best care we can provide is to honor this as much as possible. Effortlessly yielding to these changes, we have the energy to come back later when they are ready for the next thing.

Nothing Needed in Return

If we keep a tally sheet,
balancing effort against reward,
our work will surely breed resentment.

When circumstances are difficult,
we do whatever is necessary.
Neither resentment nor blame arise
because nothing is needed in return.

Our reward is independent
of the changes in external events.
It resides within our nature
and is always with us.

TAO MIND ENABLES US to look within to the true kindness and courage that emerge from the core of our being. Honoring this, we act or remain still, speak or listen, because it is an expression of who we are.

Living in this way, we are not caught up in the actions and responses of others. We can see when they are captivated by their conditioned stories. They may be afraid and resist the care that they requested an hour ago. Their reactions are not about us but reflect their internal struggle to regain a sense of clarity and safety. We do not need to change their experience; they will work their way through it in time. Witnessing this ignites our tenderness and renews our desire to be kind.

Each action is simply what we are doing in this moment. Both of us are free to gently accept what is happening now. This is our reward for living in harmony with the Tao.

We Are Missing Nothing

Our conditioned mind tells us
that we are missing something grand.
Images of delightful experiences
dance seductively in our heads.
"If only we had the time," we sigh,
"life would be so good and happy."

And then our attention returns
to the fullness of the moment.
And we realize we are here
and there is nothing else to do,
and nowhere else to be.
All the tastes and textures of life
are here to be experienced now.
There is no other time.
There is no other place.

IF ONLY ARE WORDS THAT LEAVE SORROW and frustration in their wake. These words want us to believe that there is another way to experience this season of caregiving. They point to what "should be happening" as a way of making us miserable about what is actually happening.

Let them go. There is no other time or place. There is nothing else that we should be doing to make things better. This experience was always going to contain pain and weakness, uncertainty and fear. It is the culmination of a very specific lifetime of relationships, experiences, and perspectives.

This is our life, not some diversion from it. There is not some "normal" life that is on hold for these weeks and months.

We find more ease when we do not try to give ourselves to this task and hold ourselves out of it at the same time. It will not let us "fit it in" between the important tasks of our life.

Allowing ourselves to sink fully into being present here and now, we find contentment in giving this gift of caring. In time, we discover that we would not have missed this experience for anything in the world.

81

Willingness Is the Key

When our words seem hollow
and our actions fall short
of all that we intend,
we find that we remain willing
to keep on caring.

That willingness is the key,
and simplicity is the guide.
The door of caregiving opens into freedom,
and we are able to simply be here.
That is all we have to give
and all that is ever needed.

IN CAREGIVING, AS IN ALL OF LIFE, we inevitably encounter disillusionment. The image we held of caregiving comes up against reality, of which we had very little understanding. Our persona of calm, confident caregiver is allowed to dissolve, and we find ourselves set free. This whole experience was never meant for some internal or external audience. It is life proving to us, one moment at a time, that being ourselves, just as we are, is indeed good enough.

When we release all the conditioned myths, we find that we are willing to be here. We are honored to be a humble companion on another person's journey. It is the openness of our hearts that has led us this far. It is the compassion of the Tao that will carry us through to the end.

[ABOUT THE AUTHORS]

NANCY MARTIN spent eleven years as a clergywoman with the United Methodist Church and five years as the director of volunteers for Enloe Hospice in Chico, California, where she trained and supervised volunteers working with patients and families facing end-of-life issues. For the past three years she has been the director of The Still Point, Center for Zen Practice, in Chico. She offers continuing education credits for nurses through seminars that focus on the practice of bringing compassionate awareness to the work of caregiving professionals.

WILLIAM MARTIN has worked as a research scientist, a minister, a marriage and family therapist, and a college instructor. He is now a teaching guide at The Still Point, Center for Zen Practice in Chico, California. He is the author of five books, including the classic *The Parent's Tao Te Ching*, which was picked by Oprah Winfrey to be on her "O List" of recommended books. As part of his work at The Still Point, he offers contemplative-based continuing education credits for counselors, social workers, educational psychologists, and clergy. The parents of two grown children, he and Nancy live in Chico, California.

Visit them at www.caregiverstao.com and
www.thestillpoint.com.

NEW WORLD LIBRARY is dedicated to publishing books and other media that inspire and challenge us to improve the quality of our lives and the world.

We are a socially and environmentally aware company, and we strive to embody the ideals presented in our publications. We recognize that we have an ethical responsibility to our customers, our staff members, and our planet.

We serve our customers by creating the finest publications possible on personal growth, creativity, spirituality, wellness, and other areas of emerging importance. We serve New World Library employees with generous benefits, significant profit sharing, and constant encouragement to pursue their most expansive dreams.

As a member of the Green Press Initiative, we print an increasing number of books with soy-based ink on 100 percent postconsumer-waste recycled paper. Also, we power our offices with solar energy and contribute to nonprofit organizations working to make the world a better place for us all.

Our products are available
in bookstores everywhere.
For our catalog, please contact:

New World Library
14 Pamaron Way
Novato, California 94949

Phone: 415-884-2100 or 800-972-6657
Catalog requests: Ext. 50
Orders: Ext. 52
Fax: 415-884-2199
Email: escort@newworldlibrary.com

To subscribe to our electronic newsletter, visit
www.newworldlibrary.com

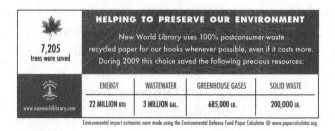

HELPING TO PRESERVE OUR ENVIRONMENT

7,205 trees were saved

New World Library uses 100% postconsumer-waste recycled paper for our books whenever possible, even if it costs more. During 2009 this choice saved the following precious resources:

www.newworldlibrary.com

ENERGY	WASTEWATER	GREENHOUSE GASES	SOLID WASTE
22 MILLION BTU	3 MILLION GAL.	685,000 LB.	200,000 LB.

Environmental impact estimates were made using the Environmental Defense Fund Paper Calculator @ www.papercalculator.org.

IDEAS IN PROFILE
SMALL INTRODUCTIONS TO BIG TOPICS

Ideas in Profile is a landmark series that offers concise entertaining introductions to topics that matter.

ALREADY PUBLISHED

Politics by David Runciman
Art in History by Martin Kemp
Shakespeare by Paul Edmondson
The Ancient World by Jerry Toner
Social Theory by William Outhwaite
Geography by Danny Dorling and Carl Lee

FORTHCOMING

Music by Andrew Gant

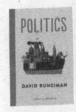
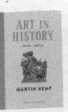
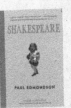
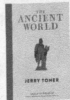